Endometriosis Diet Cookbook for Women

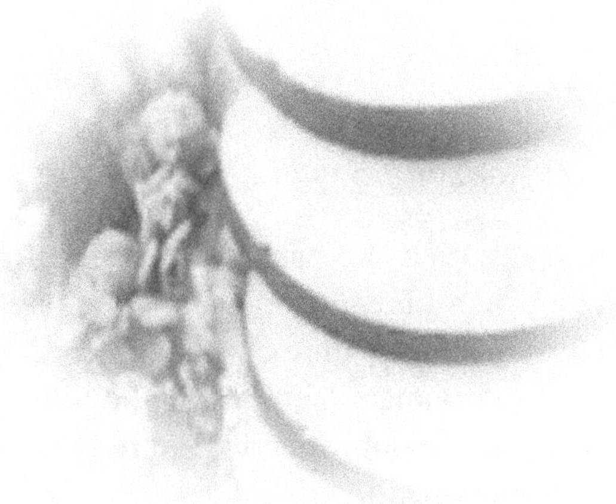

Quick and Easy Healing Recipes to manage and treat Endometriosis

David T. Salcedo

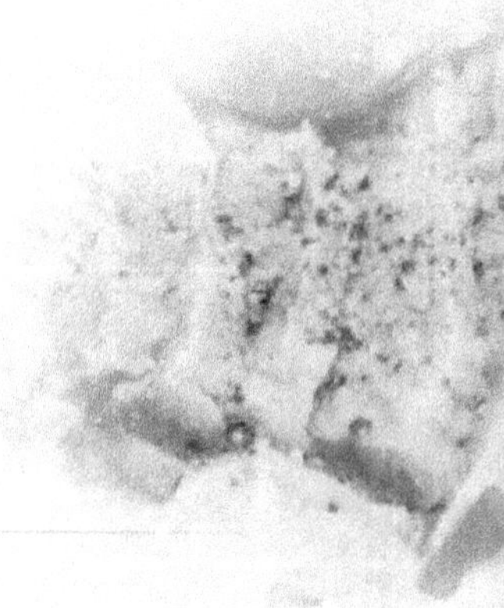

Table of Contents

INTRODUCTION

It has been a profoundly personal and inspiring experience for me to navigate and recover from endometriosis through food. In order to supplement medicinal interventions, I looked into holistic alternatives to address the obstacles posed by this chronic ailment. Through trial and error and a dedication to learning about my body, I was able to uncover the significant influence that dietary decisions can have on symptom relief and general wellbeing.

I started my path by realizing that endometriosis symptoms might be influenced by nutrition. Since the illness is inflammatory, I researched potential causes of my symptoms and spoke with medical experts to see how specific foods can make them worse or improve. The first move toward a deliberate and thoughtful approach to nutrition was this newfound understanding.

The foundation of my diet change was adopting an anti-inflammatory way of living. I purposefully gave up refined carbohydrates, trans fats, and processed foods in favor of whole, nutrient-dense foods. To help my body repair and prevent inflammation, I made it a daily practice to include an abundance of fruits, veggies, nutritious grains, and lean proteins.

After learning that omega-3 fatty acids have anti-inflammatory qualities, I started including more foods high in these vital nutrients in my diet. Walnuts, chia seeds, flaxseeds, and fatty fish became staples, providing a tasty and all-natural way to fight inflammation. Including these powerful omega-3 fatty acids improved my physical health and gave me a sense of control over my own health.

A high-fiber diet has been identified as essential for controlling endometriosis symptoms. I tried to control the condition's hormonal imbalances and bowel motions by emphasizing whole grains, fruits, vegetables, and legumes. This change in diet was crucial for maintaining overall hormonal balance as well as digestive wellness.

Recognizing my body's individuality and how it responded, I started a customized dietary adventure. By experimenting with cutting out dairy and gluten, I was able to pinpoint possible triggers and customize my diet to meet my specific requirements. During this era of self-discovery, I learned how important it was to pay attention to my body and make educated food decisions that aligned with my wellbeing.

My road to managing and recovering from endometriosis has been profoundly transforming, thanks to my commitment to nutritional mindfulness. Along with symptom relief, this approach—which incorporates nutrition—has given me the confidence to actively manage my health. I am constantly reminded of the significant relationship between the kind of life I can lead and the decisions I make in the kitchen as I develop and modify my methodology. My own life-changing experience is evidence of the healing power that comes from consciously choosing to eat a healthy diet.

What is endometriosis?

A medical disorder known as endometriosis occurs when endometrium, or tissue resembling the lining of the uterus, grows outside the uterus. Normally, during the menstrual cycle, the endometrium grows, degrades, and sheds. The displaced tissue in endometriosis behaves normally; with each menstrual cycle, it thickens, degrades, and bleeds. But this tissue gets trapped because it cannot leave the body. Adhesions, scar tissue, and cyst formation may result from this.

Types of Endometriosis

- Transient Endometriosis

The most prevalent type is marked by tiny lesions on the peritoneum, which lines the pelvic cavity.

- Deep Infiltrating Endometriosis

Deep Infiltrating Endometriosis:(DIE) is a type of the disease that affects organs like the rectum, bladder, or intestines. It involves a deeper penetration.

Causes of Endometriosis

- Menstruation in reverse

Instead of exiting the body, endometrial cells seen in menstrual blood return to the pelvic cavity.

- Biological Propensity

Your family's medical history could make you more susceptible to endometriosis.

- Immune System Impairment

The immune system may not be able to identify and get rid of endometrial tissue that has been misplaced.

- Hormonal Effects

The hormone that causes the menstrual cycle, estrogen, has the ability to encourage the development of endometrial tissue.

Symptoms of Endometriosis

- Pelvic pain

Chronic pelvic pain that frequently gets worse when a woman is menstruating.

- Dysmenorrhea, or painful menstruation

This is characterized by severe cramps that can make daily tasks difficult.

- Painful Sexual Relations

Pain or discomfort experienced during intercourse.

- Indigestion-Related Symptoms

Urinary and bowel problems, particularly during menstruating.

- Unable to conceive

Endometriosis and difficulty becoming pregnant may be related.

Prevention of Endometriosis

- Continue Living a Healthful Lifestyle

Estrogen levels and general health can be managed with regular exercise and a balanced diet.

- Early Recognition and Intervention

Timely medical intervention in response to symptoms can stop endometriosis from progressing.

- Hormone Therapies

Birth control tablets and other hormone therapies can help control symptoms and menstruation cycles.

- Operation

By removing endometrial tissue and cysts, laparoscopic surgery can alleviate discomfort.

- Pregnancy

While there are some women who report symptom improvement during pregnancy, this is not a foolproof preventive strategy.

FOODS TO EAT AND FOODS TO AVOID

Food to Eat

- Vegetables and Fruits

High in fiber and antioxidants, which can help lower inflammation.

- Complete Grains

Choose whole grains, such as quinoa, brown rice, and whole wheat, as they offer fiber and other nutrients.

- Lean Proteins

To promote general health, include lean protein sources such fish, fowl, tofu, and lentils.

- Fatty Acids Omega-3

Found in walnuts, flaxseeds, chia seeds, and fatty fish (like salmon). These may aid in lowering inflammation.

- Wholesome fats

Include foods high in unsaturated fats, such almonds, avocados, and olive oil, but in moderation.

- Spices and Herbs

Ginger and turmeric are anti-inflammatory and may be helpful.

- High-Fibre Meals

Legumes, fruits, vegetables, and whole grains can help maintain healthy digestion and control estrogen levels.

- Drinking Water

In order to maintain general health and stay hydrated, drink lots of water.

Foods to Avoid

- Processed Food

Limit your consumption of processed foods because they may have preservatives and additives.

- Sugars that have been refined

Reduce the amount of added sugar in processed snacks, candies, and sugary drinks.

- High-Grain Dairy

Some endometriosis sufferers find comfort by cutting back on or giving up high-fat dairy products.

- Gluten-free

Although not always true, some endometriosis sufferers report better results when they cut back on gluten-containing foods.

- Red Meat

Consuming too much red meat might aggravate inflammation. Instead, go for leaner forms of protein.

- Caffeine

For some people, cutting back on their caffeine intake helps assist control symptoms.

- Alcohol

Avoid drinking too much alcohol as it may aggravate inflammation.

- Soy

Despite the complexity of the association between soy and endometriosis, some people decide to consume less soy.

CHAPTER 1

Breakfast Recipes

1. Berry and Almond Smoothie Bowl

Ingredients

- Mixed berries (strawberries, blueberries, raspberries)
- Almond milk
- Greek yogurt
- Chia seeds
- Almonds (sliced)

Preparation

- Blend berries, almond milk, and Greek yogurt until smooth. Pour into a bowl.
- It should be topped with chia seeds and sliced almonds.

Nutritional Information

- Calories: 300
- Protein: 15g
- Fiber: 10g

Serving Size: 1 bowl

Preparation Time: 10 minutes

2. Quinoa Breakfast Bowl

Ingredients

- Cooked quinoa
- Fresh mango chunks
- Coconut flakes
- Greek yogurt
- Pumpkin seeds

Preparation

- Mix cooked quinoa with mango chunks and top with Greek yogurt.
- Sprinkle with coconut flakes and pumpkin seeds.

Nutritional Information

- Calories: 350
- Protein: 12g
- Fiber: 8g

Serving Size: 1 bowl

Preparation Time: 15 minutes

3. Spinach and Feta Omelette

Ingredients

- Eggs
- Fresh spinach
- Feta cheese (crumbled)
- Cherry tomatoes (sliced)
- Olive oil

Preparation

- Egg should be whisked and pour into a heated pan with olive oil.
- Add spinach, feta, and tomatoes. Cook until eggs are set.

Nutritional Information

- Calories: 280
- Protein: 20g
- Fiber: 4g

Serving Size: 1 omelette

Preparation Time: 10 minutes

4. Chia Seed Pudding

Ingredients

- Chia seeds
- Almond milk
- Vanilla extract
- Mixed berries
- Honey (optional)

Preparation

- The chia seeds, almond milk, and vanilla extract should be mixed together.
- Refrigerate overnight.
- The top should be mixed with berries and a drizzle of honey.

Nutritional Information

- Calories: 220
- Protein: 6g
- Fiber: 12g

Serving Size: 1 bowl

Preparation Time: 5 minutes (plus overnight refrigeration)

5. Sweet Potato and Kale Breakfast Hash

Ingredients

- Sweet potatoes (cubed)
- Kale (chopped)
- Eggs
- Olive oil
- Paprika

Preparation

- Roast sweet potatoes in olive oil until tender. Add kale and cook until wilted.
- The wells should be made in hash and eggs should be cracked into them.
- Bake until eggs are set.

Nutritional Information

- Calories: 320
- Protein: 15g
- Fiber: 7g

Serving Size: 1 plate

Preparation Time: 30 minutes

6. Turmeric and Ginger Smoothie

Ingredients

- Pineapple chunks
- Banana
- Greek yogurt
- Turmeric powder
- Ginger (fresh, grated)

Preparation

- Blend pineapple, banana, Greek yogurt, turmeric, and ginger until smooth.

Nutritional Information

- Calories: 250
- Protein: 12g
- Fiber: 5g

Serving Size: 1 glass

Preparation Time: 8 minutes

7. Blueberry and Oat Pancakes

Ingredients

- Oats (blended into flour)
- Eggs
- Blueberries
- Almond milk
- Cinnamon

Preparation

- Mix oat flour, eggs, blueberries, almond milk, and cinnamon. Cook as pancakes.

Nutritional Information

- Calories: 280
- Protein: 10g
- Fiber: 6g

Serving Size: 2-3 pancakes

Preparation Time: 15 minutes

8. Avocado and Smoked Salmon Toast

Ingredients

- Whole grain bread
- Avocado
- Smoked salmon
- Lemon juice
- Dill (fresh, chopped)

Preparation

- Bread should be toasted and spread mashed avocado on top.
- Add smoked salmon, a squeeze of lemon juice, and sprinkle with dill.

Nutritional Information

- Calories: 320
- Protein: 15g
- Fiber: 8g

Serving Size: 1 toast

Preparation Time: 10 minutes

9. Mango and Coconut Yogurt Parfait

Ingredients

- Greek yogurt
- Mango (diced)
- Granola
- Shredded coconut

Preparation

- Layer Greek yogurt, diced mango, and granola in a glass or bowl.
- Top with shredded coconut.

Nutritional Information

- Calories: 280
- Protein: 12g
- Fiber: 5g

Serving Size: 1 parfait

Preparation Time: 8 minutes

10. Cinnamon and Apple Quinoa Porridge

Ingredients

- Cooked quinoa
- Almond milk
- Apple (diced)
- Cinnamon
- Walnuts (chopped)

Preparation

- Mix cooked quinoa, almond milk, diced apple, and cinnamon. Heat until warm.
- Top with chopped walnuts.

Nutritional Information

- Calories: 300
- Protein: 10g
- Fiber: 7g

Serving Size: 1 bowl

Preparation Time: 12 minutes

CHAPTER 2

Lunch Recipes

1. Salmon and Quinoa Salad

Ingredients

- Grilled salmon
- Quinoa (cooked)
- Mixed greens
- Cherry tomatoes
- Cucumber
- Olive oil and lemon dressing

Preparation

- Assemble mixed greens, quinoa, grilled salmon, cherry tomatoes, and cucumber.
- Olive oil should be drizzled and lemon dressing.

Nutritional Information

- Calories: 400
- Protein: 25g
- Fiber: 8g

Serving Size: 1 plate

Preparation Time: 20 minutes

2. Vegetable Stir-Fry with Tofu

Ingredients

- Tofu (firm, cubed)
- Broccoli
- Bell peppers
- Carrots
- Snap peas
- Soy sauce and ginger marinade

Preparation

- Stir-fry tofu and vegetables in a wok with soy sauce and ginger marinade.

Nutritional Information

- Calories: 320
- Protein: 18g
- Fiber: 10g

Serving Size: 1 bowl

Preparation Time: 15 minutes

3. Mediterranean Chickpea Salad

Ingredients

- Chickpeas (canned, drained)
- Cherry tomatoes
- Cucumber
- Red onion
- Feta cheese (crumbled)
- Olive oil and balsamic dressing

Preparation

- Chickpeas, cherry tomatoes, cucumber, red onion, and feta should be combined.
- Drizzle with olive oil and balsamic dressing.

Nutritional Information

- Calories: 280
- Protein: 12g
- Fiber: 10g

Serving Size: 1 plate

Preparation Time: 10 minutes

4. Lentil and Vegetable Soup

Ingredients

- Green or brown lentils
- Carrots
- Celery
- Onion
- Spinach
- Vegetable broth

Preparation

- Cook lentils and vegetables in vegetable broth to make a hearty soup.

Nutritional Information

- Calories: 250
- Protein: 15g
- Fiber: 12g

Serving Size: 1 bowl

Preparation Time: 30 minutes

5. Whole Grain Wrap with Hummus and Veggies

Ingredients

- Whole grain wrap
- Hummus
- Spinach
- Avocado
- Shredded carrots

Preparation

- Spread hummus on a whole grain wrap and fill with spinach, avocado, and shredded carrots.

Nutritional Information

- Calories: 320
- Protein: 10g
- Fiber: 8g

Serving Size: 1 wrap

Preparation Time: 10 minutes

6. Grilled Chicken and Quinoa Bowl

Ingredients

- Grilled chicken breast
- Quinoa (cooked)
- Roasted sweet potatoes
- Broccoli
- Tahini dressing

Preparation

- Assemble quinoa, grilled chicken, roasted sweet potatoes, and broccoli.
- Drizzle with tahini dressing.

Nutritional Information

- Calories: 380
- Protein: 28g
- Fiber: 10g

Serving Size: 1 bowl

Preparation Time: 25 minutes

7. Eggplant and Tomato Stuffed Bell Peppers

Ingredients

- Bell peppers
- Eggplant (diced)
- Tomatoes
- Quinoa (cooked)
- Feta cheese
- Olive oil

Preparation

- Sauté diced eggplant and tomatoes, mix with cooked quinoa, and stuff into bell peppers.
- Top with feta and bake until peppers are tender.

Nutritional Information

- Calories: 290
- Protein: 12g
- Fiber: 8g

Serving Size: 1 stuffed pepper

Preparation Time: 35 minutes

8. Shrimp and Avocado Salad

Ingredients

- Grilled shrimp
- Mixed salad greens
- Avocado
- Cherry tomatoes
- Lime vinaigrette

Preparation

- Assemble mixed greens, grilled shrimp, sliced avocado, and cherry tomatoes.
- Drizzle with lime vinaigrette.

Nutritional Information

- Calories: 320
- Protein: 20g
- Fiber: 10g

Serving Size: 1 plate

Preparation Time: 20 minutes

9. Pesto Zoodles with Cherry Tomatoes

Ingredients

- Zucchini noodles (zoodles)
- Pesto sauce
- Cherry tomatoes (halved)
- Pine nuts

Preparation

- Sauté zoodles in pesto sauce, add cherry tomatoes, and garnish with pine nuts.

Nutritional Information

- Calories: 250
- Protein: 8g
- Fiber: 6g

Serving Size: 1 plate

Preparation Time: 15 minutes

10. Turkey and Vegetable Stuffed Acorn Squash

Ingredients

- Acorn squash (halved)
- Ground turkey
- Quinoa (cooked)
- Spinach
- Cranberries (dried)
- Cinnamon

Preparation

- Roast acorn squash, sauté ground turkey with spinach, mix with cooked quinoa, and stuff squash halves.
- Top with dried cranberries and a sprinkle of cinnamon.

Nutritional Information

- Calories: 340
- Protein: 22g
- Fiber: 10g

Serving Size: 1 stuffed squash half

Preparation Time: 40 minutes

CHAPTER 3

Dinner Recipes

1. Salmon and Asparagus Foil Packets

Ingredients

- Salmon fillets
- Asparagus spears
- Lemon slices
- Olive oil
- Garlic (minced)

Preparation

- Place salmon and asparagus on a foil sheet.
- Drizzle with olive oil, add minced garlic, and top with lemon slices. Seal and bake.

Nutritional Information

- Calories: 350
- Protein: 30g
- Fiber: 5g

Serving Size: 1 packet

Preparation Time: 25 minutes

2. Quinoa-Stuffed Bell Peppers

Ingredients

- Bell peppers
- Quinoa (cooked)
- Black beans (canned, drained)
- Corn kernels
- Tomato salsa
- Mexican cheese blend

Preparation

- Mix cooked quinoa, black beans, corn, and tomato salsa.
- Stuff bell peppers and top with cheese. Bake until peppers are tender.

Nutritional Information

- Calories: 320
- Protein: 15g
- Fiber: 10g

Serving Size: 1 stuffed pepper

Preparation Time: 40 minutes

3. Chicken and Vegetable Stir-Fry

Ingredients

- Chicken breast (sliced)
- Broccoli
- Bell peppers
- Carrots
- Snow peas
- Soy sauce

Preparation

- Stir-fry chicken and vegetables in a wok with soy sauce until cooked through.

Nutritional Information

- Calories: 300
- Protein: 25g
- Fiber: 8g

Serving Size: 1 plate

Preparation Time: 20 minutes

4. Eggplant and Lentil Curry

Ingredients

- Eggplant (cubed)
- Lentils (cooked)
- Coconut milk
- Curry spices (turmeric, cumin, coriander)
- Tomatoes (diced)

Preparation

- Sauté eggplant, add cooked lentils, diced tomatoes, coconut milk, and curry spices.
- Simmer until flavors meld.

Nutritional Information

- Calories: 320
- Protein: 15g
- Fiber: 12g

Serving Size: 1 bowl

Preparation Time: 30 minutes

5. Shrimp and Avocado Quinoa Bowl

Ingredients

- Grilled shrimp
- Quinoa (cooked)
- Avocado
- Cherry tomatoes
- Cilantro
- Lime vinaigrette

Preparation

- Assemble quinoa, grilled shrimp, sliced avocado, cherry tomatoes, and cilantro.
- Drizzle with lime vinaigrette.

Nutritional Information

- Calories: 380
- Protein: 25g
- Fiber: 10g

Serving Size: 1 bowl

Preparation Time: 25 minutes

6. Sweet Potato and Kale Frittata

Ingredients

- Sweet potatoes (diced)
- Kale (chopped)
- Eggs
- Feta cheese
- Olive oil

Preparation

- Sauté sweet potatoes and kale, pour whisked eggs over, add feta, and bake until set.

Nutritional Information

- Calories: 300
- Protein: 18g
- Fiber: 8g

Serving Size: 1 slice

Preparation Time: 35 minutes

7. Mushroom and Spinach Stuffed Chicken Breast

Ingredients

- Chicken breast
- Mushrooms (sliced)
- Spinach (chopped)
- Garlic (minced)
- Olive oil

Preparation

- Sauté mushrooms and spinach with garlic. Slice chicken breast, stuff with the mixture, and bake.

Nutritional Information

- Calories: 320
- Protein: 30g
- Fiber: 6g

Serving Size: 1 stuffed chicken breast

Preparation Time: 30 minutes

8. Cauliflower Rice Bowl with Tofu

Ingredients

- Cauliflower rice
- Tofu (extra-firm, cubed)
- Mixed vegetables (bell peppers, carrots, peas)
- Teriyaki sauce

Preparation

- Sauté tofu and mixed vegetables, add cauliflower rice, and stir in teriyaki sauce.

Nutritional Information

- Calories: 280
- Protein: 18g
- Fiber: 10g

Serving Size: 1 bowl

Preparation Time: 25 minutes

9. Tomato Basil Zucchini Noodles

Ingredients

- Zucchini noodles (zoodles)
- Cherry tomatoes (halved)
- Fresh basil
- Garlic (minced)
- Olive oil

Preparation

- Sauté zoodles, cherry tomatoes, and garlic in olive oil. Top with fresh basil.

Nutritional Information

- Calories: 250
- Protein: 6g
- Fiber: 8g

Serving Size: 1 plate

Preparation Time: 15 minutes

10. Spinach and Feta Stuffed Portobello Mushrooms

Ingredients

- Portobello mushrooms
- Spinach (chopped)
- Feta cheese
- Balsamic glaze

Preparation

- Remove mushroom stems, stuff with chopped spinach and feta, and bake.
- Drizzle with balsamic glaze.

Nutritional Information

- Calories: 280
- Protein: 15g
- Fiber: 7g

Serving Size: 2 stuffed mushrooms

Preparation Time: 30 minutes

CHAPTER 4

Snacks Recipes

1. Greek Yogurt Parfait

Ingredients

- Greek yogurt
- Mixed berries (strawberries, blueberries, raspberries)
- Granola
- Honey (optional)

Preparation

- The Greek yogurt should be layered with mixed berries and granola.
- Drizzle with honey if desired.

Nutritional Information

- Calories: 200
- Protein: 15g
- Fiber: 4g

Serving Size: 1 parfait

Preparation Time: 5 minutes

2. Hummus and Veggie Sticks

Ingredients

- Hummus
- Carrot sticks
- Cucumber slices
- Bell pepper strips

Preparation

- Dip vegetable sticks into hummus.

Nutritional Information

- Calories: 150
- Protein: 5g
- Fiber: 8g

Serving Size: 1 serving

Preparation Time: 5 minutes

3. Trail Mix with Nuts and Seeds

Ingredients

- Almonds
- Walnuts
- Pumpkin seeds
- Dried cranberries
- Dark chocolate chips

Preparation

- Mix all ingredients in a bowl.

Nutritional Information

- Calories: 250
- Protein: 8g
- Fiber: 5g

Serving Size: 1/4 cup

Preparation Time: 2 minutes

4. Cottage Cheese and Pineapple Bowl

Ingredients

- Cottage cheese
- Fresh pineapple chunks
- Chia seeds

Preparation

- Combine cottage cheese with pineapple chunks and sprinkle with chia seeds.

Nutritional Information

- Calories: 180
- Protein: 15g
- Fiber: 3g

Serving Size: 1 bowl

Preparation Time: 5 minutes

5. Apple Slices with Almond Butter

Ingredients

- Apple slices
- Almond butter

Preparation

- Spread almond butter on apple slices.

Nutritional Information

- Calories: 160
- Protein: 4g
- Fiber: 6g

Serving Size: 1 apple's worth of slices

Preparation Time: 3 minutes

6. Chia Seed Pudding with Berries

Ingredients

- Chia seeds
- Almond milk
- Mixed berries
- Maple syrup (optional)

Preparation

- The chia seeds should be mixed with almond milk and refrigerate overnight.
- It should be Topped with mixed berries and a drizzle of maple syrup if desired.

Nutritional Information

- Calories: 220
- Protein: 6g
- Fiber: 10g

Serving Size: 1 bowl

Preparation Time: 5 minutes (plus overnight refrigeration)

7. Roasted Chickpeas

Ingredients

- Chickpeas (canned, drained)
- Olive oil
- Smoked paprika
- Garlic powder

Preparation

- Toss chickpeas with olive oil, smoked paprika, and garlic powder. Roast until crispy.

Nutritional Information

- Calories: 180
- Protein: 7g
- Fiber: 6g

Serving Size: 1/2 cup

Preparation Time: 30 minutes

8. Edamame and Sea Salt

Ingredients

- Edamame (steamed)
- Sea salt

Preparation

- Steam edamame and sprinkle with sea salt.

Nutritional Information

- Calories: 120
- Protein: 11g
- Fiber: 6g

Serving Size: 1 cup

Preparation Time: 10 minutes

9. Cucumber and Tzatziki Bites

Ingredients

- Cucumber slices
- Tzatziki sauce
- Cherry tomatoes
- Fresh dill (optional)

Preparation

- Top cucumber slices with tzatziki sauce, a cherry tomato, and fresh dill if desired.

Nutritional Information

- Calories: 90
- Protein: 3g
- Fiber: 2g

Serving Size: 1 serving

Preparation Time: 5 minutes

10. Avocado and Tomato Rice Cakes

Ingredients

- Rice cakes
- Avocado
- Cherry tomatoes (sliced)
- Everything bagel seasoning

Preparation

- Spread mashed avocado on rice cakes, top with sliced cherry tomatoes, and sprinkle with everything bagel seasoning.

Nutritional Information

- Calories: 160
- Protein: 2g
- Fiber: 5g

Serving Size: 2 rice cakes

Preparation Time: 5 minutes

CHAPTER 5

7 Days Meal Plan

Day 1

Breakfast: Berry and Almond Smoothie Bowl

Lunch: Salmon and Quinoa Salad

Dinner: Salmon and Asparagus Foil Packets

Snack: Hummus and Veggie Sticks

Day 2

Breakfast: Quinoa Breakfast Bowl

Snack: Trail Mix with Nuts and Seeds

Lunch: Vegetable Stir-Fry with Tofu

Dinner: Quinoa-Stuffed Bell Peppers

Day 3

Breakfast: Spinach and Feta Omelette

Snack: Apple Slices with Almond Butter

Lunch: Mediterranean Chickpea Salad

Dinner: Chicken and Vegetable Stir-Fry

Day 4

Breakfast: Sweet Potato and Kale Breakfast Hash

Snack: Edamame and Sea Salt

Lunch: Whole Grain Wrap with Hummus and Veggies

Dinner: Sweet Potato and Kale Frittata

Day 5

Breakfast: Turmeric and Ginger Smoothie

Snack: Cucumber and Tzatziki Bites

Lunch: Shrimp and Avocado Salad

Dinner: Cauliflower Rice Bowl with Tofu

Day 6

Breakfast: Blueberry and Oat Pancakes

Dinner: Tomato Basil Zucchini Noodles

Lunch: Pesto Zoodles with Cherry Tomatoes

Snack: Roasted Chickpeas

Day 7

Breakfast: Mango and Coconut Yogurt Parfait

Snack: Chia Seed Pudding with Berries

Lunch: Turkey and Vegetable Stuffed Acorn Squash

Dinner: Mushroom and Spinach Stuffed Chicken Breast

CHAPTER 6

Conclusion

Through the transformational power of diet, we have discovered a world of nourishment that extends well beyond the act of eating in our journey to manage and heal from endometriosis. This book has served as a mentor, a friend, and an inspiration to people navigating the complex terrain of their health.

Let's consider the human body's resiliency and the significant influence that conscious, nourishing choices can have on our overall wellbeing as we draw to a close. The recipes presented here are more than just a compilation of ingredients; they serve as evidence that the foods we choose to eat can have a significant impact on our recovery process.

Let us say goodbye to these pages with a feeling of empowerment and a dedication to the continuous practice of self-care. May the healing flavors continue to permeate the lives of those seeking comfort and strength, and may the lessons learned here find a home in every kitchen.

Keep in mind that this is merely a chapter in your continuous journey toward resilience and health, not just a book. Cheers to seeing every day as a chance to appreciate all that life has to offer and to treat the body with the respect it so richly deserves. I hope your path is one of healing, vigor, and celebration of the amazing, life-changing power of your own decisions.

THANKS FOR READING